How to Go Natural Without Going Broke

Crystal Swain-Bates

How to Go Natural Without Going Broke
ISBN 978-1-939509-03-1

Goldest Karat Publishing
340 S Lemon Ave #1077
Walnut, CA 91789

Disclaimer: Product prices in the book are accurate at the time of
writing. Vendors may change their prices at any time.

First Edition

Table of Contents

PREFACE

How is it that going natural became synonymous with going broke?

Since cutting off my relaxed hair and going natural in 2010, I have become a magnet for relaxed and natural heads alike sharing their reasons for or against doing the same. To date, one of the most striking reasons I heard for not going natural—and part of the impetus for writing this book— was from a woman who simply said, "It costs too much." This caught me off guard, because many natural-haired women have shared the exact same answer as their reason for going natural in the first place: they were tired of spending money on relaxers. I asked the woman what it was about being natural that cost so much, and she explained that natural hair "just requires too much stuff," from special shampoos to oils to curl enhancers to different combs, etc., all designed specifically for natural hair.

Once the initial shock wore off, I thought about what she had said and realized that while natural hair does not cost a lot of money to maintain, there certainly is a perception that it does. If you go to your nearest beauty supply store or peruse the ethnic hair care section of your local Walmart or Target, you are certain to find endless shampoos, conditioners, hair oils, butters, and puddings for kinks, curls, and otherwise natural or unrelaxed hair. Natural hair bloggers and YouTubers are constantly reviewing the latest and greatest products for natural hair, and it seems as though nearly every product they try is the holy grail. Natural hair forums are filled with product junkies, women who are addicted to purchasing hair products and are willing to allocate a sizeable percentage of their paychecks to products that are solely aimed at helping them wash, style, or condition their hair. While this might not be an issue for women who have enough disposable income to make such purchases, what becomes of those who don't? I'm talking about the broke college students, the unemployed, the underemployed, the single parents, and anyone else who just might have more important things to spend her money on than natural hair products. Are they destined to live "unnappily" ever after?

Have you been dissuaded from going natural because you think you can't afford it? Are you a hair product junkie in need of an intervention? Are you one deep conditioner or curly pudding away from being homeless? Could you benefit from learning ways to save money on your natural hair?

If you answered "maybe" or "yes" to any of the above questions, this book is for you! Going natural is only as expensive as you make it. This book, written by a recovered hair product junkie, is aimed at changing the perception of the costs required to grow and maintain natural hair by providing money-saving tips and tricks that will help women go natural without going broke.

The 10 Hair Commandments for Going Natural Without Going Broke

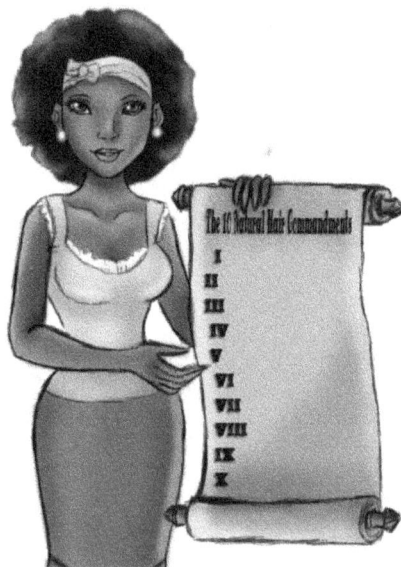

1. Know Thy Hair

The first and most important golden rule for going natural without going broke is to get to know your hair. Sure, you know what color it is, you know the general shape of your coils, kinks, or curls, and you know the length. If you follow the various hair typing systems, you might even know if the size of your curls classifies you as a 3b or a 4a. None of these details is particularly important in the grand scheme of things. Going natural is kind of like starting a new relationship. If the only thing you know about the person is that he or she is tall, slender, and brown-skinned, you really haven't gotten very far. It's not until you learn people's likes, dislikes, and how they respond to various situations that you really know them. It might sound a little crazy, but you have to think of your hair in similar terms. What ingredient does your hair like the most? Are there any specific ingredients that your hair doesn't care for? For example, some people have protein-sensitive hair, while others can't use products with glycerin because it makes their hair feel sticky and dry. Another important thing to know before you start purchasing hair products is what your hair looks like naked, meaning freshly washed with no products added. I wouldn't be surprised if many natural women have no clue what their naked hair looks like. We get so used to using our leave-in conditioners and gels that it never occurs to us to see what our hair looks like without them. You may be shocked to discover that your hair actually curls just fine without using that expensive curl-enhancing product. Why is this important? The more you know about your hair, the better choices you can make when buying hair products, because you can avoid wasting money on products with ingredients that your hair doesn't like.

Get to know what your hair is like without products, and use that knowledge to help you decide the kind of products you actually need to purchase.

2. Know Thy Ingredients

Just as you read the ingredients labels on food items, you should do the same with your hair products. Labeling laws require manufacturers to list ingredients on the label in descending order of predominance by weight. This is important, because if you are purchasing a shea butter hair cream and shea butter is listed near the end of the ingredients list, you might want to put that product back on the shelf, because it contains a pretty small amount of shea butter. By the same token, if you pick up a moisturizing hair conditioner and the first ingredient on the label is water, you should probably keep that one in your cart since all moisturizing conditioners should contain a significant amount of water. Take the same approach when it comes to ingredients your hair doesn't like. If you know that your hair doesn't respond well to glycerin, mineral oil, or protein, don't purchase products with these ingredients listed high up on the ingredients list. Contrary to popular belief, you don't have to completely avoid all products with less desirable ingredients, but you definitely want to make sure they are lingering somewhere near the end of the ingredients list.

Ingredients aren't the only thing you want to pay attention to when looking at product labels. Watch out for the slick marketing of products as "all-natural," "botanical," "herbal," or any of the other buzzwords companies slap on a product to justify charging more for it. Currently, regulatory law does not define these terms; therefore, any company can label its products as such without needing to meet any real requirements. Unlike the buzzwords listed above, the word "organic" cannot be thrown around willy-nilly. It actually does have a regulatory definition, which states that products bearing the U.S. Department of Agriculture Organic label must contain a minimum of 95% of organic ingredients. However, products with the phrase "Made with Organic Ingredients" on the label are only required to contain a minimum of 70% of organic ingredients.

3. Thou Shalt Skip the Brand Names

In the last decade, a brand-name natural hair market has emerged. However, for many of the expensive products designed for women with natural hair, the price of the product reflects the name on the label rather than the quality of the product itself. In order to go natural without going broke, you have to recognize that for nearly every expensive natural hair care product, there is a cheaper alternative. Are you willing to pay more for the name brand when you could purchase the cheaper drugstore equivalent without sacrificing quality? As is typically the case when pitting brand names against less expensive drugstore brands, if you look closely you may find that they have the same or very similar ingredients, and the only difference is the price. Unless you make enough money to buy that Versace-labeled jar of curly pudding without a second thought, you should stretch your dollars by seeking out alternative products that serve the same purpose but lack the high price tag.

4. Thou Shalt Know where to Go

In terms of saving money, shopping for products for your natural hair is much like shopping for groceries. You know that Kroger has the best prices for cheese, Publix has the cheapest milk, and Whole Foods has the cheapest … well, nothing! Joking aside, you should have a general sense of where to find the best prices on products for your natural hair. Don't assume that the price of natural hair products at Target will be the same as at Walmart, Sally's Beauty, Amazon, or your local drugstore. Surprisingly, sometimes the price variations are quite substantial. This book will be a valuable resource to guide you to the best money-saving deals online and at your local stores.

5. Thou Shalt Simplify Your Regimen

I cannot overstate the importance of creating and sticking to a simple hair regimen. This alone is a major way to avoid breaking the bank on your natural hair. If you have spent any time perusing natural hair blogs or watching natural hair videos on YouTube, you have probably encountered women with overly extensive regimens that require the use of "fifty-'leven" products. Despite what you may have seen online, you need only a few products to maintain your natural hair, many of which you can make yourself. The beauty of having a simple regimen is that it saves money and makes it easier to determine how your hair responds to each product. If you begin experiencing dry and brittle hair but your regular routine requires the use of eight different products, how will you ever be able to pinpoint the culprit? It's quite simple: you won't.

6. Thou Shalt Seek Double Threats

Try to limit your hair product purchases primarily to what I like to call double threats: items that serve at least two purposes. When it comes to saving money, it makes more financial sense to purchase products that serve multiple purposes than to buy individual items that are good for only one thing. This book highlights numerous double threats (as well as some triple threats) that not only are hair-friendly but can be used to moisturize the skin or whip up a delicious meal; it includes products that are both edible and, well, "headable."

7. Thou Shalt Do It Yourself

One of the most effective ways to go natural without going broke is to break your reliance on hair stylists and learn how to do your hair yourself. Now, don't get me wrong, I'm not trying to put hair stylists out of business. I think we all love getting our hair done. But let's face it, when your money is looking funny, getting your hair done is a luxury, not a necessity. You shouldn't have to cut into your grocery money to get your hair done, but you also shouldn't have to look busted if you can't make your monthly hair appointment. Make it a personal goal to perfect at least three different hair styles within your first few months of being natural. If you want to boost your savings, take things a step further by learning how to trim your own hair. You'll save money and avoid the way-too-common experience of having a scissor-happy stylist give you a haircut rather than the trim you requested. The nice thing about doing your hair yourself is that in addition to saving money, you save the gas you would have spent driving to a stylist and the time you would have spent waiting to be seen. Finally, you gain peace of mind from knowing that your kinks and curls are in safe hands: yours!

8. Thou Shalt Think outside the Natural Hair Box

Natural hair looks very different from straight, untextured hair. While each person's hair is indeed unique, at the end of the day it's still just hair, and it can respond positively to many of the popular products on the market even if they aren't specifically labeled as being for natural kinks, curls, or coils. In fact, you don't even have to use products from the ethnic hair care aisle. That's right! Companies such as L'Oreal, Neutrogena, Tresemme, and Herbal Essences make excellent products that work for multiple hair textures, including natural hair. I wince when people tell me that they threw away all their old hair products as soon as they went natural. First of all, throwing away hair products is a no-no when it comes to saving money, because many products can easily be modified to make them work better for your hair by diluting them with water, adding oils, or mixing them with other products. Second, rather than throwing unwanted hair products away, you should "freecycle" them by visiting a site such as www.freecycle.org, which helps you give them away to people or organizations who can reuse them. Until you can think outside the natural-hair box when purchasing products, you will miss out on opportunities to acquire wonderful natural-hair-friendly products at discount prices.

9. Thou Shalt Share with Care

While you may be excited to share the newfound knowledge you have gained from this book and other natural hair resources with friends and family, don't be surprised if they don't always share your enthusiasm for your new practices. Many of the tips in this book fall outside the traditional norms for black hair care and require a certain level of open-mindedness, an ability to think outside the box. These virtues are inherent in many natural-textured women, as evidenced by their decision to go natural in the first place. However, your coworkers, family, and friends may be shocked and appalled to find out what products you are using in your hair—and they may be quite vocal about it. Don't be discouraged by negative comments. Just make a mental note not to share your hair practices with those who are critical of them. Rather than wasting energy explaining why you do what you do, let your hair growth and increased bank account do the talking!

10. Thou Shalt Be Patient

Growing out your natural hair is a journey, not a race. No hair product, no matter how expensive, will make those beautiful kinks, coils, or curls grow out of your head any faster than the average speed of half an inch per month. So just relax and enjoy the natural hair ride!

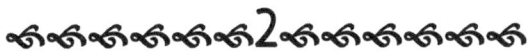

2
Repurpose Your Goods

This chapter focuses on how to repurpose common household goods and use them to benefit your natural hair. Repurposing your goods is Earth- and wallet-friendly, as it gives a new purpose to items you might otherwise have thrown away.

Reuse Your Bottles

Spray bottles, while an essential component of a natural woman's toolkit, are an unnecessary expense. Why pay for a new bottle when you probably have many under your bathroom sink? After using up your favorite sprayable styling product (or pouring out the contents of your least favorite sprayable product!), rinse the bottle thoroughly and *voilà!* You have a new spray bottle to use as you please. Refill it with a mixture of water and conditioner, aloe vera juice and water, or your favorite combination of products, to use on your hair as a daily misting spray. If the bottle is small enough, leave it empty and carry it in your purse. Simply refill with water as needed during the day for a hair touch-up on the go.

The same principle holds true for product applicator bottles: either reuse the bottles of the hair products you currently own or just make your own.

If you are really in a DIY mood, you could also repurpose mustard bottles by washing them out and using them as product applicators. The best thing about a mustard bottle is that its skinny nozzle will help you get products directly onto your scalp. If you have thick hair, this is a great way to get shampoo to your roots. Just be sure to label the mustard bottle so that you (or an unsuspecting member of your family) don't accidentally end up squirting shampoo onto your turkey sandwich. You've been warned!

Use a T-shirt to Dry Your Hair

Did you disobey the age-old rule about not washing reds and whites together? If one of your white cotton T-shirts decided to cross the color line to mingle with the "coloreds," leaving you with a pink garment, don't throw it away! Repurpose the ruined T-shirt as a hair-drying tool. Drying your natural curls with a T-shirt is gentler than using a towel, reduces frizz, and helps keep your curl pattern intact.

There are lots of different ways to wear the T-shirt turban. This is how I wear mine: put the T-shirt on normally and then begin to take it off. Once you get the neck of the shirt around your head and hairline, stop and tie the loose ends of the shirt into a knot, or just gather them up with a scrunchie. Need a visual? Search YouTube for "T-shirt head wrap."

Use Straws for Rollers

Regular plastic drinking straws, rather than perm rod rollers, can be used to achieve a long-lasting curly look, appropriately called a "straw set." To achieve this style, section your hair into 1/4 inch to 1/2 inch sections. Take a small amount of hair in one of the sections, comb it through, apply setting lotion, and wrap the hair around a straw. Secure the hair to the straw using a bobby pin and move on to the next bit of hair in that section. Repeat this process until your entire head has been completed. Let hair

air dry or sit under a dryer. Do not remove the straws until the hair is 100% dry; otherwise, your style will be frizzy. The final look of your straw set will be determined by the length and thickness of the straws. The general rule is that the longer the straw, the longer the curls, and the thicker the straw, the looser the curls.

No More Tension Headaches

Got a run in your stockings? Don't throw them away! Recycle them by turning them into a custom-fit hair accessory that's perfect for making a puff. Regular ponytail holders are often too small to comfortably hold thick natural hair. Save money and prevent a tension headache by cutting off the leg of a stocking and using it as a headband. It's stretchy and you can control the tightness of the stocking around your head. Or you can cut off the top band of a knee-high and use that as a headband. Experiment with different techniques until you find one that works best to keep your hair in place.

Ditch the Shower Caps

Given all the deep conditioning treatments that natural-haired women do (or should do), shower caps are an ongoing purchase, and despite how inexpensive they are, the cost can add up over time. Sure, you could reuse your shower caps to save money, but you will have to wash them out thoroughly each time to prevent the remnants of last week's henna treatment from getting mixed in with this week's deep conditioner. I'm not really the wash-out-my-shower-cap kind of girl, so I choose to save money by repurposing a common item, the plastic grocery bag. Unless you religiously carry a reusable shopping bag with you everywhere, you are bound to accrue a few plastic grocery bags with each trip to the store. What better way to make use of them than to substitute them for shower caps? Using grocery bags as shower caps is an economical and earth-friendly way to recycle. Besides, depending on how much hair you have, regular shower caps might not be large enough. Before I discovered this alternative, I was using two shower caps each time I conditioned—twice as expensive as just using one! Even the woman with the largest Afro in the world could fit all her wet hair into a grocery bag. To rock this look, place your conditioned hair inside the plastic bag and then tie the handles of the bag against your forehead or secure them with a claw clip. Some things are more easily seen than read, so visit the blog at www.mochamoolah.com if you need a visual.

I know some of you are shaking your heads right now, thinking that this sounds and probably looks ridiculous. You are absolutely right! The good news is that you aren't trying to win any beauty contests; your goal is to focus on easy ways to save money in the comfort of your own home. So don't knock it 'til you rock it!

If you can't get down with the grocery bag thing, you can use saran wrap instead. However, it's not as economical, since you don't get saran wrap for free.

Toothbrush Hairbrush

For many women, using a toothbrush to style natural hair is common knowledge. From slicking back your edges with gel to laying down your baby hair to channel your inner Chilli, the toothbrush is an excellent addition to your natural hair toolkit. If you brush your hair infrequently, it is a gentle, cost-effective alternative to a travel-sized brush or even a regular-sized brush. Since the toothbrush is smaller than your regular hair brush, you can use it to carefully slick back the hair in hard-to-reach areas, such as behind your ears.

Here are a few more ways you can use the toothbrush you've added to your toolkit:

- Dip it in shampoo to clean your scalp when wearing braids or cornrows.

- Wet the toothbrush, dip it in baking soda, and gently scrub your scalp to remove dead skin cells and product buildup.

- Use a soft toothbrush and shampoo to clean your combs and hairbrushes.

- Use it to clean out the vent on your blow dryer.

- Use it to brush gel between your cornrows when they start to fray.

Wine Cork Hair Rollers

Here's one for the winos … I mean, the wine enthusiasts out there. The next time you finish off a bottle of wine, save the cork. Once you've saved enough corks, you can use them as hair rollers. Sure, they aren't as soft as foam rollers, but they sure are softer than regular plastic rollers. Believe it or not, braids or two-strand twists set on corks make a beautiful twist and curl! Simply wind one small braid or twist around a cork and secure with a bobby pin. Repeat until your entire head is done.

Oh Bobby!

Bobby pins are a natural diva's best friend. Many natural hair styles, from buns to frohawks to pompadours, require bobby pins to keep them in place. For some reason, however, these little suckers are hard to keep track of, which may mean that you find yourself buying a new pack every month. Save money and keep your breath fresh by using an empty TicTac container as a bobby pin holder.

Please Pass the K-Y

Personal lubricant doesn't only work wonders "downstairs"; it can also work wonders upstairs. Just as you apply a makeup primer to your freshly washed face, you can apply K-Y liquid to freshly washed natural hair to seal in moisture and reduce frizz. Don't worry about the effect of K-Y on your hair; the product is primarily composed of water and glycerin, both of which help the hair and skin to maintain moisture. Besides, if it's safe to use in your most sensitive area, it's definitely safe for your hair as well—unless, of course, your hair is glycerin-sensitive. Some women actually use K-Y as a face moisturizer, so this is a product that will give you a lot of bang for your buck. The ingredients in K-Y are very similar to the ingredients in Curly Hair Solutions Curl Keeper, a product that provides frizz control and curl definition for curly hair.

If you want to avoid the embarrassment of your friends and family seeing your huge container of K-Y on the bathroom counter, transfer it to an unmarked, judgment-free container.

ക‑ക‑ക‑ക‑ക‑ക‑ക3ക‑ക‑ക‑ക‑ക‑ക‑ക

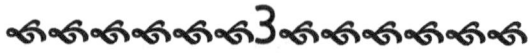

Do It Yourself

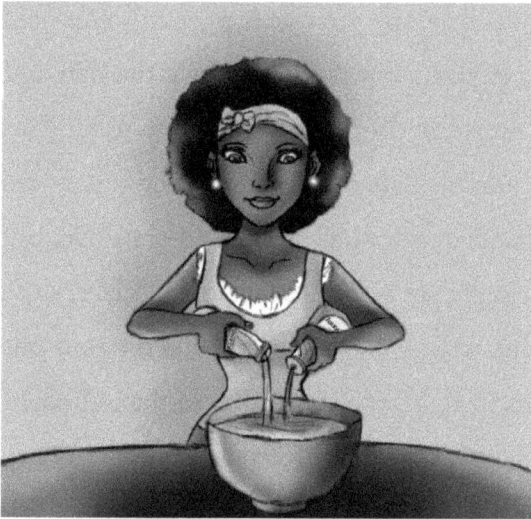

*Darren Hardy, the publisher of Success magazine, once wrote,
"What's in your head determines what's in your wallet." This
rings true in the matter of going natural without going broke.
One of the most gratifying ways to save money on your hair is to
take (hair) matters into your own hands and embrace the art of*

doing it yourself. Learning how to style your natural hair and make or customize your own products is one of the most empowering things you can do for yourself. Over time, your newfound skills will bring immeasurable financial savings.

Learn to Style Your Own Hair

Can't afford hair school? Think again. In the past two years, YouTube has become a virtual school of cosmetology taught by hundreds of natural-haired "fro-fessors." From the comfort of your home, you can learn hundreds of styling techniques, including:

- How to grow out your relaxer and transition to natural hair;

- How to properly wash and detangle natural hair with minimal breakage;

- How to achieve popular natural hair styles such as two-strand twists, braidouts, buns, frohawks, puffs, and roller sets;

- How to straighten your natural hair with minimal damage;

- How to trim your natural hair;

- How to color your natural hair.

Look for women whose natural hair is a similar length and texture to your own, for the most easily duplicated results. For example, my hair is very thick and coily with a lot of shrinkage, so I tend to watch more styling videos by women with similar hair because I can usually get my hair to look like theirs by following their directions verbatim. I still watch and appreciate other hair videos, but I get the best styling results from watching my hair twins. Beware when selecting videos to watch, as not all YouTube "fro-fessors" are created equal! If a YouTube fro-fessor doesn't have a head of healthy-looking natural hair, you might want to think twice about following her techniques and advice. If you are new to natural hair and can't easily determine which fro-fessors are safe to watch, YouTube offers some helpful features, such as viewer comments and likes and dislikes for each video. If a hair-straightening video has more dislikes than likes and comments that criticize the fro-fessor's straightening techniques, for example, this would be a pretty good indicator that you need to keep looking. Many of the popular YouTube personalities document their hair growth over time, lending them more authority because they can prove that their natural hair practices work. Keep in mind that these YouTubers and bloggers are experts on their natural hair, not yours, so use discretion when deciding to purchase items they recommend. Remember, you may not experience similar results.

Here are some of my favorite natural hair YouTubers:

Naptural85:
http://www.youtube.com/user/Naptural85

SimplYounique:
http://www.youtube.com/user/SimplYounique

African Export:
http://www.youtube.com/user/AFRICANEXPORT

007NewNew:
http://www.youtube.com/user/007newnew

Natural Chica:
http://www.youtube.com/user/Nikkimae2003

BeautifulBrwnBabyDol:
http://www.youtube.com/user/BeautifulBrwnBabyDol

Kimmaytube:

http://www.youtube.com/user/kimmaytube

Fusion of Cultures:

http://www.youtube.com/user/FusionofCultures

Mahogany Knots:

http://www.youtube.com/user/mahoganyknots

Alicia James:

http://www.youtube.com/user/aliciajamesmusic

MsVaughnTV:

http://www.youtube.com/user/MsVaughnTV

Get Wiggy with It

If you want to switch up your look without the cost and time associated with going to a hair stylist, consider wearing a natural-looking wig as an economical alternative. Wigs can look incredibly natural if you know how to wear them, and at around twenty bucks for a synthetic one, they won't break the bank. I occasionally get the urge to wear a roller set, but I'm not patient enough to do it myself and I don't want to pay to get my hair done, so I simply wear my roller-set-style wig. When I'm in the mood for straight hair but don't want to run the risk of getting heat damage, I wear a natural-looking kinky-straight wig instead of paying a stylist to straighten my hair. The beauty of wearing a wig to change up your look is that you don't have to pay a stylist every time you want a look that you can't achieve on your own. Plus, you can keep your own tresses safely protected under the wig and just remove it when you get home.

The website "Wigs for Natural Hair" at www.wigsfornaturalhair.com is a wonderful resource for women who are searching for wigs that look similar to their natural hair. The site includes information on numerous kinky-straight, kinky-curly, and Afro-style wigs and has informative articles about using wigs as a protective style while growing out or transitioning to natural hair.

Let's Get Steamy

Steaming is an easy and effective way to maximize the benefits of your deep conditioning treatments and give your hair a boost of moisture. The process of steaming opens the hair cuticle to allow conditioner to penetrate more easily, making your curls super-defined, soft, and easy to detangle. Don't own a hair steamer and can't afford to purchase one? No steamer, no problem! Here are two simple and economical ways to get the benefits of steam without the high price tag of buying your own steamer.

Do you have a gym membership? If so, after getting your workout in, double-dip by heading to the steam room to give your curls a free steam treatment. Liberally apply the conditioner of your choice to your damp hair and wrap your hair in a hair towel, or just enter the steam room with your naked hair for the greatest benefit. Steam your hair for ten to fifteen minutes, rinse with cool water, and then apply a smoothing leave-in conditioner to seal the cuticle.

If you don't have access to a steam room, here's a technique you can do at home:

1. Saturate your hair with the conditioner of your choice and cover the hair with a plastic shower cap. Soak a large face cloth or small hand towel in water, wring it out so that it isn't dripping wet, place the towel in a gallon-sized plastic bag, and put in the microwave. Heat the towel in the unsealed bag for thirty-five seconds or until hot.

   Note: The moisture will keep the towel from

catching fire in the microwave, but don't go overboard by leaving it in longer than sixty seconds at a time.

2. Remove the towel from the bag, being careful not to burn yourself. Once you can comfortably do so, wring most of the water out of the towel and wrap it around the plastic cap on your head. Now cover your entire head with one more plastic cap, a grocery bag, or saran wrap. Leave on until the towel is no longer hot. Reheat the towel to repeat, if needed. The heat from the hot, moist towel will help open the follicles in your hair, resulting in better absorption of the conditioner you have applied.

3. Rinse hair with cool water to seal the cuticle.

Make Your Own Leave-in Conditioner

Leave-in conditioners are an unnecessary expense when you are on a limited budget. Thick natural hair will suck up quite a lot of leave-in conditioner, especially if the product is very watery; making your own will save you from this frequently recurring purchase. Choose your favorite conditioner, put a squirt or two into a clean, empty bottle, and fill the rest of the bottle with water. Leave enough room to be able to thoroughly blend the mixture by shaking the bottle. A ratio of 30% conditioner to 70% water may provide the best results for your hair, but you can adjust the ratio as you see fit. No need to use exact measurements, just eyeball it. Use a spray bottle if you plan on making a very watery leave-in conditioner, as this will make it easier to apply the product without spilling.

Bentonite Powder

If your curls, coils, or kinks are starting to look dull and lack their usual pop, a bentonite powder treatment may be just what the hair doctor ordered. Mixed with water, this powdered volcanic clay, also known as Fuller's earth, is an excellent natural hair cleanser and conditioner.

Here is how to make a cleansing hair mask from bentonite powder: Slowly add enough water to the clay to form a creamy mixture with the consistency of pancake batter. If you like, add honey or conditioner to make the mask more moisturizing. Apply the treatment to wet hair and cover with a plastic cap. Leave the mask on for fifteen to twenty minutes and then rinse thoroughly. Follow up with a light conditioner and rinse again. When you think all the clay has been washed out, rinse one more time just to be sure. Once the mask is removed, you should be left with clean, soft, moisturized hair that has super-defined curls. Save a little bit of the mixture and apply it to your face for a pore-cleansing, spa-quality facial!

Tip: Be sure to rinse the mask out of your hair before it dries. Otherwise, it will be very difficult to remove. This is not a treatment you want to do overnight.

You can also make your own bentonite hair wash using this recipe:

½ cup bentonite clay
¼ cup extra virgin olive oil
¼ cup apple cider vinegar
½ cup aloe vera juice
A wooden or plastic spoon—metal and bentonite don't mix!

Mix the bentonite powder and apple cider vinegar until the lumps have dissolved. Add aloe vera juice and stir until the mixture has the consistency of cake batter. Slowly add the extra virgin olive oil until the mixture reaches the desired thickness.

To apply the mud wash, clip your wet hair into sections and saturate it with the mixture. Once all the sections are done, mist hair lightly with water and cover it with a plastic cap. Wash out after about thirty minutes. Take care not to let the mixture dry in your hair.

Apply leftover mud wash to your face and body.

Oils

Every few months it seems as though someone discovers some new, exotic oil that supposedly works miracles on your hair and, consequently, takes a miracle to be able to afford. Remember when emu oil blew up and became the "it" product of the year? Well, emu oil comes from the fat of the Australian emu bird, and, unfortunately, the bird must be killed in order to extract it. Now, I want shiny, moisturized hair just as much as the next person, but I don't want it that bad! Argan oil, which is more humane since it comes from the fruit of the Moroccan argan tree, is currently one of the most popular oils on the block. Despite the popularity contest, many of the more common oils, such as olive oil, coconut oil, jojoba oil, and grapeseed oil, are extremely beneficial to natural hair. They are also less expensive and easier to find in stores. Let's examine these oils in closer detail.

Virgin coconut oil. Coconut oil is widely considered to be a miracle worker for women with natural hair. Have you ever heard of those six-in-one oils that do everything from moisturizing your hair to softening your skin? Well, coconut oil is like a twenty-five-in-one oil: it can be used for the skin, for the hair, to aid in weight loss, for cooking, as a deodorant, as a makeup remover … the list goes on and on. Because of the small size of its molecules, coconut oil is one of the few oils that actually penetrate the hair shaft, adding moisture and shine to the strands. Besides moisturizing the hair, it has anti-fungal properties that help prevent and treat dandruff, so you don't need to continue purchasing expensive, chemical-laden dandruff shampoos. Contrary to what its name implies, coconut oil is an oil only at temperatures above around 76°F (assuming that you keep the temperature in your home around 72°F in the wintertime, 76°F is a few degrees warmer than your typical room temperature). You can store coconut oil in the refrigerator if you want it to remain completely solid until you melt it in your hands, but I prefer storing it in a pantry, because it stays soft enough for me to easily scoop some out with my spoon. Coconut oil has an average shelf life of two years, making it a highly cost-effective purchase, especially when compared to oils that go rancid within just one year. To receive the greatest benefits, try to purchase an edible cold-pressed, unrefined coconut oil; it will have undergone less processing than a refined oil, whose taste, fragrance, color, and texture will have been changed by the refining process. Popular brands include Nutiva, Nature's Way, Garden of Life, and Tropical Traditions. You should be able to purchase a 15-oz. jar of coconut oil for under ten dollars.

So, how do you use coconut oil in your hair? Here are a few ideas:

- If shampoo leaves your hair feeling stripped and dry, try using coconut oil as a pre-shampoo treatment by applying it to your hair one hour before washing.

- If your hair is braided or twisted, melt a quarter-sized amount of coconut oil by rubbing it between your hands. Then rub it into your hair to keep your hair moisturized and shiny. If you are rocking a twist-out, the oil will reduce frizz and leave you with a healthy-looking, non-greasy shine.

- To use coconut oil as a deep conditioner, apply it liberally to your hair after shampooing and cover with a plastic cap for one hour. Rinse. Your hair will be soft and tangle-free.

- To make your curls pop and shine, mix coconut oil with your gel and apply it on top of a leave-in conditioner.

- As an added bonus, coconut oil is an excellent alternative to ordinary cooking oil. Try sautéing sweet potatoes in coconut oil for a healthy and flavorful twist. You can also spread a little coconut oil and honey on your toast for breakfast.

Olive oil. While you may be more accustomed to pouring olive oil into your skillet than onto your hair, you probably won't even require a trip to the store to purchase this natural ingredient. Olive oil has been used for centuries to alleviate dryness, improve elasticity, and restore shine and strength to hair. It contains large amounts of the antioxidant Vitamin E, which prevents hair loss and contributes to hair growth by improving the health of the scalp. This ultra-hydrating, vitamin-rich oil may be too heavy for frequent usage by those with finer hair, but it works very well on medium-to-coarse-textured hair.

Here are a few ways to incorporate olive oil into your hair regimen:

- Liberally apply olive oil directly to your hair to add shine;

- Beef up the moisturizing properties of your regular conditioner by adding a few tablespoons of olive oil to it;

- Make your own hot oil treatment by heating olive oil in a microwave-safe container until the oil is warm to the touch. Apply the oil to your hair and cover with a shower cap. I like to tie a scarf or sweater around my head so that it traps my body heat and absorbs any drips.

Jojoba oil. Pronounced "ho-ho-buh," this is actually a non-greasy liquid wax, rather than an oil. Putting liquid wax in your hair probably doesn't sound very appealing, so I will refer to it as an oil. Jojoba oil's molecular structure is nearly identical to that of the natural oils found in the hair and skin, allowing it to be quickly absorbed. Jojoba oil strengthens the hair follicle and shaft, helps promote a healthy scalp, and reduces hair loss by clearing clogged pores. Jojoba oil can be applied directly to the hair and is good for all hair textures, particularly for fine hair that is weighed down by heavier oils. Jojoba oil can be purchased from Walgreens, GNC, and the Vitamin Shoppe.

Grapeseed oil. Pressed from grape seeds and rich in Vitamin E, this lightweight, non-greasy oil can be used for hot oil treatments, moisturizing hair, and, in a crunch, as a heat protectant, since it can withstand heat up to 450°F. As an added bonus, when regularly applied to the scalp it can prevent itchy scalp and dandruff.

Apple Cider Vinegar

Commonly referred to simply as ACV, apple cider vinegar is good for more than just dressing salads. Used as a hair rinse, this household staple removes product buildup, detangles the hair, and seals the cuticle, leaving your curls smooth and shiny.

Here's a simple recipe for an apple cider vinegar hair rinse you can use once a week to maintain shiny, healthy hair. This rinse has the added benefit of restoring your hair's natural pH balance and soothing itchy scalp and dandruff.

- For oily to normal hair, mix one part apple cider vinegar with four parts distilled water. For dry hair, use a mixture of one part apple cider vinegar to six parts distilled water.

- After shampooing or conditioner washing ("co-washing") your hair, pour the apple cider vinegar rinse over your hair and massage it into your scalp. Rinse with warm water, then seal your cuticles with cool water.

You might feel like a walking salad at first, but the smell will disappear once your hair dries.

Aloe Vera

Aloe vera juice, a mineral-rich ingredient found in many products designed for natural hair, is a useful addition to your arsenal of raw ingredients. Aloe Vera is a natural hair conditioner, strengthener, and pH balancer that will leave your hair frizz-free, silky, and smooth.

- Mix one-quarter cup aloe vera gel with olive oil to make a natural hair conditioner.

- Mix aloe vera juice and your favorite oil in a bottle and use it as a daily hair moisturizer.

Baking Soda

You may already know that the little orange box of Arm & Hammer® baking soda is good for more than just deodorizing your fridge. It has a plethora of uses in personal hygiene and general household maintenance. If your hair stops responding to your normal products or routine, or if it looks dull or feels coated, you might need to clarify it. Baking soda is an excellent natural hair clarifier; it helps remove the residue left behind by styling products, so your hair is cleaner and more manageable. How often you need to clarify depends on the products you use in your hair. If you have been using a lot of gel or non-water-soluble silicones, or if your hair has been in a braided or twisted style for a prolonged period of time, you may need to clarify to remove product buildup that cannot be removed by shampoo or co-washing alone.

There are several benefits to using baking soda as a clarifier. First, it's cheap and easy to obtain. Second, you can control the strength of the clarifier by adjusting the amount of baking soda you use. Since baking soda changes the pH of the hair (don't worry, most things do, including water), you don't want to make the solution too strong, so stick to using only a tablespoon or two until you determine the best water-to-baking-soda ratio for your hair.

Here is a quick and easy way to make a clarifying baking soda hair treatment:

Spoon no more than two tablespoons of baking soda into an empty water bottle (extra points for recycling), add warm water and give the bottle a few good shakes, until the baking soda is fully dissolved.

Tip: Make sure you use warm water for this, as—trust me— pouring a bottle of cold water over your head in the shower is not the most pleasant experience.

In the shower, soak your hair with water from the showerhead and then pour some of the baking soda "shampoo" over your head. Gently massage the mixture into your scalp, concentrating on getting it clean. Once you are done, thoroughly rinse the mixture out of your hair and immediately follow up with an apple cider vinegar rinse to return your hair to its normal pH. Skipping this step will leave the cuticles of your hair raised and susceptible to damage, so don't overlook it!

Honey

This sweet nectar deserves a place in both the kitchen and the bathroom. It is a natural humectant, which means it attracts and retains moisture. Honey will draw moisture from the air and lock it into your natural hair. It also has antimicrobial properties, making it a gentle and effective cleanser.

So, how do you apply honey to your hair? The most important thing you need to know is that you should not apply the honey directly to your hair, as it will literally leave you with a sticky mess on your hands. Instead, try one of the following recipes to add honey to your natural hair routine:

- To make a spray leave-in conditioner, add honey and hot water to a spray bottle and shake hard until the two ingredients are mixed together. The amount of honey and water you use will depend on the size of your bottle. As a general rule, use about one cup of water for every tablespoon of honey.

- To make a moisturizing hair treatment, heat about one-half cup of honey for fifteen seconds or until it is warm to the touch, and mix it with one-quarter cup of olive oil. Work a small amount at a time through your wet natural hair until it is fully coated, focusing on the ends of your hair. Cover hair with a shower cap and leave on for thirty minutes. Remove shower cap. Shampoo or co-wash well and then thoroughly rinse your hair.

- Apply the leftover honey-and-oil mixture as a face mask. It will trap and seal in moisture, leaving your skin soft as a baby's you-know-what!

Yogurt

Are you getting enough protein in your hair diet? A protein deficiency can make natural hair brittle and weak, resulting in hair loss. Depending on how often you style with heat, dye your hair, or use rough grooming techniques—all of which can wear down the protein bonds in your hair—you may need to do a protein treatment about once every four to six weeks. Packed with hair-strengthening protein, yogurt is a cheap and easy way to make a protein treatment that will help restore strength to your hair. Naturally high in lactic acid, yogurt will help to shine and smooth tangled hair, making it easier to comb. Don't worry, the lactic acid won't damage your curls.

Of course, there is no need to spend money on an expensive protein treatment. Here are a couple of ways to incorporate yogurt into your natural hair routine to give your curls a protein-packed punch:

- Massage room-temperature plain yogurt into your hair to smooth tangles and give your curls added shine.

- To make a protein-rich deep conditioner, mix six tablespoons of Greek yogurt with four tablespoons of honey and one teaspoon of an oil of your choice.

- Can't find Greek yogurt? Mix one egg white, one-half cup of plain, full-fat yogurt, and two tablespoons of your favorite oil. Apply to damp hair and rinse out after thirty minutes.

Bananas

Are your bananas more brown than yellow? Don't waste money throwing those overripe bananas away. Make them a part of one of your hair cocktails. Bananas are incredibly rich in vitamins and natural oils that help soften the hair and maintain natural hair's elasticity. When using real bananas, you must puree them using a blender or food processor; otherwise, you will spend the next few days cursing my name as you pick banana pieces from your hair. If you don't have a way to puree the bananas on your own, don't worry. Just pick up a one-dollar jar of banana baby food the next time you go to the grocery store.

To make your own banana deep conditioner, mix one large pureed banana or one jar of baby food with four tablespoons of your favorite oil and two tablespoons of honey. Apply to damp hair and let sit for 30 minutes under a shower cap, grocery bag, or saran wrap. Rinse thoroughly and style as usual.

Coconut Milk

Coconut milk is another cheap, all-natural product that leaves natural hair soft, moisturized, and strengthened. Loaded with protein and fatty acids, coconut milk mixed with honey makes a deep conditioning treatment you can use as a pre-poo or a cheap conditioner. Look for cans of coconut milk in the Asian food aisle of your grocery store. To use it, don't shake the can; just use a can opener to remove the metal top and then skim the upper fatty portion of the coconut milk off the surface. This is the part you want to use. (To make sure that the fatty portion will rise to the top, you can refrigerate the can the day before you use it.) Mix with a few tablespoons of natural hair-friendly additives such as honey, olive oil, or even your favorite conditioner.

Note: If your hair is protein-sensitive, skip this conditioner.

You won't use the entire can of coconut milk, so be sure to refrigerate the remainder and use it within a few days to avoid spoilage. To get the most bang for my buck, I usually use coconut milk in my "mixtress" creations when I cook coconut curried chicken. Since my recipe only calls for about three-quarters of the can, instead of throwing the rest away I use it on my next shampoo day.

If you don't cook with coconut milk, another way to avoid wasting the remainder is to divide it into two or three quart-size plastic storage bags and freeze them. Alternatively, you could pour the leftover coconut milk into an ice-cube tray and freeze it. Then just defrost your coconut milk ice cubes as needed.

Beef Up a Conditioner

If you have a conditioner that's just not moisturizing enough, don't throw it away. Instead, beef that conditioner up by customizing it to meet your hair's particular needs. The next time you plan to condition your hair, pour the amount you want to use into a bowl. Then let your inner mixtress take charge. Add a few tablespoons of your favorite oil and two teaspoons of honey, stir, and watch your new and improved conditioner appear before your eyes. In order to prevent any bacteria growth, it's best to whip up these remixed conditioners in a separate container right before use, rather than adding the ingredients directly to the bottle of conditioner.

Stretch an Expensive Conditioner

The same principle applies to products you really like. If you purchased a high-end conditioner and you want to stretch it as far as it can go, you can add your favorite oils and honey to it in a separate container to stretch it out and make it last longer. This will save you money, since you will have to purchase it less frequently.

Tip: Be sure to properly store your mixtress creations. To play it safe, unless you are adding preservatives to your mixtures, store your homemade mixes in the fridge and use them within one week.

Maintain Your Drain

What do you get when you mix oils, shampoo, conditioner, soap, and natural hair? A recipe for a clogged drain. Many of our favorite products for natural hair include heavy oil-based ingredients that can wreak havoc on your drains. Every time you wash your hair in the shower or kitchen sink, you are mixing hair and oil, which create drain-clogging hair balls that can be a beast to remove. Unless you are a big fan of picking foul-smelling, soap-scum-covered hair out of your drain, preventive maintenance is the name of the game.

Before purchasing one of the numerous unclogging chemicals on the market, try one of the following methods of preventing and clearing hair-clogged drains:

- Avoid spending money on costly plumbing repairs by limiting the frequency and severity of bathtub clogs. The cheapest way to avoid drain strain is to keep your hair out of the drain in the first place. Purchase a cheap hair-catching drain cover from a hardware store, Walmart, Lowes, or Home Depot to prevent your hair from going down the drain.

- As a preventative measure, carefully pour a pot of boiling water down the drain every week to wash away potential clogs.

- Once a month, pour one-half cup of baking soda down a clogged drain, then follow it with one-half cup of vinegar. Wait five minutes and flush the drain with boiling water.

- For the already sluggish drain, add one-quarter cup of baking soda to the vinegar. The foaming reaction may help unclog the drain. Allow the mixture to work for thirty minutes, then flush with boiling water.

- If your drain is already clogged, pour one cup of bleach into the hair-clogged drain and flush with hot water after thirty minutes.

- Alternatively, if you'd like to avoid using harsh chemicals in your drains, I highly suggest purchasing a Zip-It drain unclogger. At around three dollars, this long piece of plastic is a smart addition to your natural hair toolkit. Its hair-grabbing teeth will allow you to remove hair easily from your drain by yourself without paying for an expensive plumber. Pick up a Zip-It at Walmart, Home Depot, Lowe's, ACE Hardware, True Value, Do It Best, Walgreens, Rite Aid, or Canadian Tire. Check out the customer videos of the Zip-It in action at http://zipitclean.com/ to see how it works.

❧❧❧❧❧❧4❧❧❧❧❧❧❧
Shopping

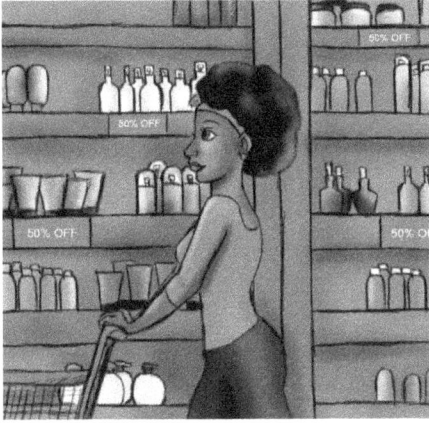

*By now you have learned how easy it is to make your own
products for your natural hair. For those items you'd still like to
purchase from a store, use the following tips to save money.*

Don't Impulse Buy

Have you ever gone to the grocery store planning on buying a carton of eggs and a gallon of milk, and walked out with a jar of coconut oil and a 32-oz. ounce bottle of conditioner? The next time you head to the store, try one of these tips to decrease the chances of making an impulse buy:

1. Skip the health and beauty section. Seriously! Just avoid it completely. If you are supposed to be buying eggs and milk, you need to stick to the periphery of the store where they keep those items instead of wandering down the center aisles, where you can easily get distracted by shiny objects.

2. If you skip tip number one because you just can't go to the store without taking a peek at the hair section, and you end up finding something you'd like to buy, make yourself leave it on the shelf until you've finished the rest of your shopping. The goal is to put distance between yourself and the product, so that either you forget to purchase it or you decide you don't want it after all.

3. Instead of buying the item, take a picture of it—
   making sure the price is visible in the picture—and
   then do some research online to read reviews and
   compare prices at the online retailers. Like tip
   number two, this will put distance between yourself
   and the product, and chances are you won't end up
   buying it after all.

4. If you are a self-certified hair product junkie, enter
   the store with only enough money to purchase the
   items on your shopping list. Knowing that you have
   immediate access to only ten dollars in cash will
   make it pretty hard for you to purchase items that
   aren't on your shopping list.

The Problem with Sales

Saving money is good. Saving money by buying products
you didn't need or want until you saw them on sale is bad.
Ask yourself if you were already thinking of buying that
item before you entered the store. When you see a
hundred-and-fifty-dollar hair steamer on sale for 50% off,
don't focus on the percentage of the reduction. Instead,
look at the product in terms of its actual price—in this case,

seventy-five dollars plus tax. Remember, just because something is affordable, that doesn't mean you need to buy it. In fact, if you see a product on sale, you will always end up saving more money by not buying it at all.

Shopping Buddy

When you are about to make an impulse buy, have a few people you can call to get their take on whether or not you really need the item. My shopping buddy has always been my mom. I call her when I'm about to make what I know is an unnecessary purchase, and she does the same when she's in a similar position. It works! Sometimes, hearing a few words of reason is all it takes to drown out that voice in your head telling you to "Buy, buy, buy!"

Do Your Research

If you are out shopping and you spot a hair product you've never seen before, don't just grab it and throw it in your cart. Look it up, right there in the store. Research potential hair-related purchases thoroughly, especially if they are non-refundable. The wonderful thing about this smartphone age is that information is always right at your fingertips, so you have no reason not to do your research before buying something.

These days, I don't buy much of anything without looking it up first. If I can't find at least one review online, I think long and hard about whether or not I want to purchase the item. With thousands of natural hair bloggers and product reviewers on the web, you can rest assured that someone has written something about nearly every natural hair product that exists.

Hold Out for a Sale

Late November through early January is the best time to score big deals on natural hair products, particularly on Black Friday, Cyber Monday, and Christmas. Many of the popular natural hair companies, including Miss Jessie's, Karen's Body Beautiful, Oyin Handmade, Qhemet, and Carol's Daughter, have major sales during the holiday season, offering deals such as free gifts with purchase or— my personal favorite—buy one, get one free. This is the perfect time to stock up on your favorite high-end products, as well as products from smaller companies that specialize in natural hair products.

This is one of the only times during the year that I make any major hair purchases. I like handmade natural products, but I don't like paying handmade prices, so I use the discounts offered during the holiday season as an opportunity to stock up on items for which I refuse to pay full price. For the products you use often, buy enough of them during a sale, if possible, to last you until the next sale. It usually takes me nearly six months to finish an entire container of a styling product, since I don't use any of them exclusively, so I only have to purchase two containers to last all year.

Before purchasing, always be sure to find out the shelf life of the product. There's no point in stocking up on something only to have it go bad before you have a chance to finish using it.

Take It Back

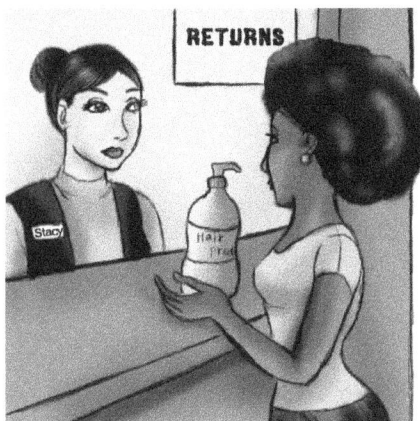

Have you ever purchased a hair product that promised you the world but did nothing for your curls? Did you stick it in the hair product graveyard under your bathroom sink, leaving it to join the other curl puddings, conditioners, and stylers that failed you in the past? If so, from this point forward keep all the receipts from your hair product purchases. The next time you buy a product that your hair doesn't like, take it back to the store. Since drugstores don't usually offer testers for their products, it can be hard to judge whether or not you like a product until after you purchase it and get it home; however, many major drugstores and beauty product retailers will let you return items you didn't like, usually within thirty to sixty days of purchase. Save money by restricting your purchases to stores that have a lenient return policy. When in doubt, before you purchase anything at your local store just ask the clerk what the return policy is. Here are the return policies of four different beauty retailers, current at the time of writing:

CVS wants you to *"be 100% happy or receive 100% money back on any beauty products. If you're dissatisfied for any reason, you can return the beauty product (opened or unopened) along with your receipt or invoice to any CVS/pharmacy store. We'll refund the full purchase price—no questions asked! To return the item by mail, call Customer Care at 1-888-607-4CVS (1-888-607-4287). We'll work to ensure that both your return and credit refund are processed accurately."*

Rite Aid drugstore has a 100% Risk-Free Beauty Guarantee, which states, *"Any opened or used beauty product of any brand name can be returned for a full refund when accompanied by a receipt. Beauty categories subject to the guarantee are skin care/depilatories, sun care, bath/soap, hair care (shampoo, conditioner, styling and professional), hair color, cosmetics, ethnic beauty aids, fragrances, cosmetic organizers and personal care appliances."*

The return policy of the large beauty retailer **Ulta,** which sells drugstore brands as well as higher-end salon products, states, *"ULTA is dedicated to bringing you an unparalleled shopping experience from start to finish. If you are not completely satisfied with a product for any reason, just send it to the Ulta.com Returns Center for a refund. You may also return it to your local Ulta store for a refund, exchange or in-store credit."*

According to **Walmart's** website, *"If you bought something at a Walmart store and need to return or exchange it, you can take it back to any Walmart store, not just the one where it was purchased,"* and, *"For most items, we accept returns within 90 days after purchase."*

Pay in Cash

From this point forward, pay for all your hair products in cash rather than by credit or debit cards. Having to physically hand over your hard-earned cash is a lot harder than simply swiping a card. It will instantly make you think twice about what you are purchasing. And, as a money-saving bonus, paying in cash will prevent you from paying interest on your hair care purchases.

Do the Math

Don't be afraid to pull out your calculator and figure out the cost per ounce for products you are thinking of purchasing. Why pay $4 for an ounce of shampoo when you can buy the big 16-oz. bottle for only $12? That's $4 per ounce versus $1.33 per ounce. As a real-life example, let's look at Carol's Daughter's Hair Milk. The 8-oz. hair milk costs $20, while the 2-oz. trial size costs $9. You don't even have to pull out your calculator to see that the 2-oz. product is horribly overpriced. Although your frugal side might feel more comfortable spending $9 rather than $20, instead of the measly two ounces of product you might as well spring for the larger size and call it a day. Besides, will two ounces even be enough to truly determine whether your hair likes the product or not? Sometimes we get so excited to see natural hair products for under ten dollars that we buy two or three of them, and ultimately we spend the same amount of money, or more, as we would have spent had we just bought the product we really wanted in the first place.

Avoid Travel Sizes

Instead of buying travel-size hair products, buy a set of travel bottles so that you can fill them with your own products. Better yet, do what I do. The next time you stay at a hotel, repurpose the free hotel toiletries they give you by emptying the bottles and thoroughly rinsing them out. These bottles usually hold about one ounce and are the perfect size and shape for travelling with shampoo, conditioner, leave-ins, etc. Best of all, you don't have to spend a dime on the bottles.

Buy in Bulk

While most local retailers sell the 8 ½-oz. "holy grail" Giovanni Direct Leave-In Conditioner for $7.99, the liter (33 ounces) can be purchased online at massagewarehouse.com for only $12.99. Let me break that down for you: at $7.99, the 8 ½-oz. bottle costs 94 cents per ounce, while the $12.99 liter is only 39 cents per ounce. That's a cost difference of almost 250%. If you bought four of the 8 ½-oz. bottles, you would be spending $31.96 for 34 ounces when you could have spent only $12.99 for 33 ounces.

Save money by buying hair products in bulk and splitting them with a friend. For example, if you use EcoStyler gel in your daily hair routine, you could save money by purchasing the 5-lb. jar and splitting it with a friend. This is cheaper than buying it in smaller quantities. You each end up with two and a half pounds of gel for approximately the same price as the 32-oz. jar.

Stick with It

Once you find products that work really well in your natural hair, stop buying new ones. Yes, I know this is much more easily said than done, but just hear me out. How many times have you purchased a new leave-in conditioner or a new gel when you already had perfectly good ones at home? Often, when we see new products or hear good things about ones we haven't used, our curiosity gets the best of us and we just have to try them. Once we try that new product, we push the old one to the side. Later on, we hear about yet another one we'd like to try, and the cycle continues. Funnily enough, sometimes in this "lather, rinse, repeat" cycle of trying out new hair products, we eventually end up circling right back to the products we loved in the first place and ask ourselves why we ever stopped using them to begin with. Unless your favorite products are expensive and you are looking for cheaper alternatives, try to avoid unnecessarily spending money testing out new products when you already have ones at home that you love. You know the saying: If it ain't broke....

Group Buy

If you live in a city that has little or no supply of products that work well with your natural hair, and you find yourself ordering these products online as a result, consider group buying as an opportunity to save money on shipping. If you have friends in your area who have natural hair, chances are that they are having the same problem as you. So give them a call before placing your next order online. You never know, they may want to order something as well. Group buying will help you save money because you can split the cost of shipping with your friends or, in many cases, receive free shipping once you've met the minimum purchase amount, which may happen more easily when you've combined the orders of two or more people.

Look for Product Twins (or Cousins)

I have alluded to this in an earlier section: most of the expensive hair products have a cheaper alternative. As the natural hair care market continues to expand, so will the range of knockoffs you can purchase to save money. Here are some examples:

1. The Denman brush works well to detangle naturally curly or kinky hair, but at around $9 a pop, you may want to save money by purchasing one of its knockoff cousins. The popular company Goody makes a nine-row brush that is nearly identical to the ever-so-popular Denman and is less than half the price. The company Conair makes a seven-row brush that is also very similar to the Denman. Visit your local CVS or Walgreens to find either one of these Denman lookalikes.

2. Curlformer knockoffs. Want to get heatless curls on your natural hair, but don't want to spend $60-plus at Sally's for the Curlformers Salon Kit? Search ebay for the MajicLeveragCurlformers knockoff, at less than $20 for the entire set.

3. Giovanni's Tea Tree Triple Threat Invigorating Conditioner and Trader Joe's Tea Tree Tingle Conditioner are definitely kin. While they may not be brothers, they are definitely first cousins. The following list is a comparison of these conditioners, with ingredients in bold type representing matches between the two:

Trader Joe's Tea Tree Tingle Conditioner: **water, tea tree oil, peppermint oil, eucalyptus oil, nettle oil, thyme oil,** birch leaf oil, **chamomile oil,** clary oil, **coltsfoot leaf, yarrow oil,** mallow, **horsetail oil,** soybean protein, **cetyl alcohol,** Vitamin E, trace minerals, **citric acid,** sodium hydroxymethylgycinate, grapeseed.

Giovanni's Tea Tree Triple Threat Invigorating Conditioner: **aqua (purified water) with melaleucalternifolia (tea tree) leaf oil, menthapiperita (peppermint) leaf extract, eucalyptus (eucalyptus officinalis) oil, thymus vulgaris (thyme) extract, urticadioica (nettle) extract, tussilagofarfara (coltsfoot) flower extract,** salvia officinalis (sage) leaf extract, rosmarinusofficinalis (rosemary) leaf extract, lavandulangustifolia (lavender) leaf extract, **equisetum arvense (horsetail) extract, chamomillarecutita** (chamomile) flower extract, achelleamillefolium (yarrow) extract, cetyl alcohol, stearyl alcohol, glycerin, brassicamidopropyldimethylamine, panthenol, cetrimonium chloride, cetearyl alcohol, hydroxypropyl guar, behentrimoniummethosulfate, menthol, polysorbate 60, citric acid, disodium EDTA, ethylhexylglycerin, phenoxyethanol, fragrance with essential oils.

Once you get past the long scientific names on Giovanni's label, you can see that many of the ingredients, particularly the first few, are the same. As we've already mentioned, the ingredients are always listed in order of concentration, from highest to lowest. The most active ingredients in these two conditioners are the same, which means that the Trader Joe's conditioner is a close knockoff of the Giovanni brand. In fact, it has been speculated online that the Tea Tree Tingle Conditioner is Trader Joe's store version of the Giovanni product.

4. Just can't bear the thought of dropping $22 for an 8-oz. container of Miss Jessie's Curly Pudding? Head to Walgreens and pick up an 8-oz. jar of Softee's Signature Curli Q Fondue for only $3.99.

Let's compare the Curli Q Fondue ingredients to Miss Jessie's Curly Pudding. Ingredients in bold type represent matches between the two products:

Softee's Signature Curli Q Fondue: **water**, petrolatum, **glycerin, shea butter,** cetyl alcohol, **triethanolamine, carbomer,** panthenol , **aloe barbadensis leaf extract, jojoba seed oil , avocado oil,** polyquaternium-7, **peg-12 dimethicone, ethylhexylmethoxycinnamate, fragrance,** citric acid, methylchloroisothiazolinone, methylisothiazolinone, **ext. violet 2.**

Miss Jessie's Curly Pudding: **water**, praffinum liquidum (mineral oil), **glycerin, fragrance, triethanolamine, carbomer, peg-12 dimethicone,** dipropylene glycol, silk amino acids, **aloe barbadensis leaf extract, avocado oil, shea butter,** sweet almond oil, **jojoba seed oil,** macadamia seed oil, oleth-5, **ethylhexylmethoxycinnamate,** disodium EDTA, DMDM hydantoin, **ext. violet 2.**

While the two products are not exact duplicates of each other, there are way too many similarities between them not to produce comparable results. At less than one-fifth the cost of Miss Jessie's Curly Pudding, Softee's Curli Q

Fondue offers a fantastic alternative that won't break the bank.

5. III Sisters of Nature, a Georgia-based company, offers a range of hair styling products that are free of alcohol, silicones, petrolatum, mineral oil, parabens, and other ingredients you might be trying to avoid. At the time of writing, the company does not have a website and their products are not sold online. However, you can find them at certain Kroger grocery store locations.

The III Sisters of Nature Curling Gelo is a duplicate of Kinky Curly Curling Custard. See their Facebook page for more information: http://www.facebook.com/pages/III-Sisters-of-Nature/175665912510970

Shop Your Discount Retailers

Ross, Marshalls, and TJ Maxx are known for their great deals on clothing, purses, and housewares, but have you ever taken a look at the hair care section? Did you even know they had a hair care section? Different locations carry different items, so you may need to visit a few stores to see what deals you can find. For example, many TJ Maxx and

Marshalls locations carry the 33.8-oz. bottles of Giovanni shampoos and conditioners for only $12.99. Brands such as Joico, Chi, Nature's Gate, Abba, EO, Twisted Sista, and even Carol's Daughter have been spotted at these stores. When it comes to Ross, I always have good luck finding pretty hair accessories for bargain prices—so much so that I have changed their slogan from "Dress for Less" to "Tress for Less." All three stores usually carry heavily discounted 100% silk scarves for less than ten dollars, and if you straighten your hair frequently, check the shelves for ceramic flat irons at huge discounts. If you live in the United Kingdom, don't fret. TJ Maxx exists there as well, but with a slight variation in the name: TK Maxx. While UK ladies have the luxury of ordering products online from www.tkmaxx.com, the website for TJ Maxx doesn't currently offer this convenience.

Dollar Stores

Don't skip the health and beauty section of the various dollar stores in your area, such as Family Dollar, Dollar General, and Dollar Tree. For an example of the type of natural-hair-friendly products many dollar stores stock, just take a look at the link http://www.dollardays.com/wholesale-ethnic-bath-and-body.html.

The next time you drive by one of these stores, don't be afraid to go in and see what they have. You never know, you might find a product you normally purchase, for only half the cost of what you usually pay. Keep an eye out for any of the following items: Fruit of the Earth Aloe Vera Gel, honey, disposable shower caps, bobby pins, elastic hair bands, and hair flowers.

Big Lots

Big Lots is a retail chain in the United States that sells closeout and overstock merchandise. Many Big Lots sell food, housewares, books, toys, and health and beauty items. This is a good place to purchase olive oil, hair accessories, and hair products. Because of the nature of the closeouts business, the catch is that the inventory of these stores changes frequently and without notice, so you never know what you will find. Furthermore, once an item is gone, it may be gone forever. So if you find a good deal on a product you need, purchase it immediately, because there is no guarantee the store will ever have that item in stock again.

Shop Your International Grocery Stores

Top international supermarket chains often specialize in providing Asian foods, but they also carry a variety of African, Indian, Caribbean, and Hispanic products. Whereas avocados usually cost over a dollar at regular grocery stores, the normal price at ethnic supermarkets is sometimes as low as forty cents. Besides avocados, you can often find olive oil, coconut milk, and beauty products such as beeswax (for slicking back your edges) and rosewater (to hydrate your hair) at low prices.

If you aren't familiar with any international grocery stores in your area, do a Google search using phrases such as "international supermarket," "ethnic grocery store," "Hispanic grocery store," or "Asian grocery store."

Two examples of international grocery stores with locations throughout the U.S. are Grand Mart, which has stores in Virginia, Maryland, Washington, D.C., North Carolina, and Georgia (their website http://www.mygmart.net/ is in

Korean), and H Mart, which has stores in Georgia, New York, New Jersey, Massachusetts, Pennsylvania, Maryland, Virginia, Illinois, Texas, California, Colorado, Washington, and Oregon, Ontario, Canada, and London. Visit http://www.hmart.com/ for more information.

If you don't want to make a separate trip to an international grocery store, visit the ethnic food section of your regular grocery store. Some CVS locations have a section in which they stock products aimed at their Hispanic customers, where you can usually find rosewater and other hair-healthy items at reasonable prices.

Try Before You Buy

Some stores have product testers available for popular natural hair products, allowing you to do a strand test on your own hair to see how it reacts. I don't often see people taking advantage of this, but believe me, having the ability to smell a product, feel its texture, and apply it to a curl or two can really help you decide whether it's the right product for you. How many times have you purchased a natural hair product and excitedly ripped it open once you got home, only to discover that you hate the smell or it doesn't do anything for your hair? Sephora currently has Carol's Daughter products available as testers; I admit I recently spent about thirty minutes trying out different products on different pieces of my hair to help me decide which ones, if any, I wanted to buy. What's nice about Sephora is that if you ask nicely, they will give you a small sample of the product to try at home. Some Whole Foods stores will also provide samples of selected products in their hair care section. As my mom always tells me, if you ask, you have everything to gain and nothing to lose. So whenever possible, try products before you buy them. If you have friends with natural hair, do product swaps with them so that you get to test out different products before buying them yourself.

Drugstore Cheapies but Goodies

One source of hair product bargains is none other than your local drugstore, such as CVS, Walgreens, Ricky's, or Rite-Aid. These stores often have "buy one, get one free" sales and offer bonus bucks on products that work wonders on natural hair. Many K-Mart, Walmart, and Target stores also carry natural hair care products and accessories. The selection will differ depending on where you live.

Many products that have received rave reviews from women with natural hair can be purchased easily and cheaply at a local store. As a recovered product junkie, I can say from personal experience that the products on the following list worked well for me and were well worth their reasonable costs. Prices are subject to change.

Shampoos/Conditioners

Creme of Nature Argan Oil Moisture and Shine Shampoo, 12 oz. for $6.49 at Walgreens;

Giovanni Shampoos and Conditioners, 8½ oz. for $7.99 at Walgreens, or cheaper in larger sizes at Ross, Marshalls, TJ Maxx, or http://www.massagewarehouse.com/;

Trader Joe's Tea Tree Tingle Conditioner, 16 oz. for $3.99 at Trader Joe's;

Yes to Carrots/Yes to Cucumbers conditioners, 16.9 oz. for $8.49 at Walgreens;

Nature's Gate conditioners, 18 oz. for $5-$8 at Whole Foods or CVS, or for $4.49 at www.vitacost.com;

Herbal Essences Hello Hydration or Long Term Relationship Conditioner, 10 oz. for $3.99 at Walmart;

Tresemme Naturals Nourishing Moisture Conditioner, 25 oz. for $5.99 at Walgreens;

Beautiful Textures Tangle Taming Conditioner, 12 oz. for $6 at Walmart;

VO5 Silky Experiences Conditioner, 15 oz. for $.99 at Walmart.

Deep Conditioners

Silk Elements Mega Cholesterol Conditioning Treatment, 20 oz. for $4.79 at Sally Beauty;

Hollywood Beauty Cholesterol, 20 oz. for $2.99 at your local beauty supply store;

Organic Root Stimulator Hair Mayonnaise, 16 oz. for $10.99 at Sally Beauty.

Leave-in Conditioners

Cantu Shea Butter Leave In Conditioning Repair Cream, 16 oz. for $4.99 at Walgreens;

Kinky Curly Knot Today, 8 oz. for $11.99 at Target;

Giovanni Direct Leave-in Conditioner, 8½ oz. for $7.99 (the best value is $12.99 for 33 oz. at http://www.massagewarehouse.com. Note: The large sizes of the Giovanni Direct Leave-in are a rare find at local stores);

Taliah Waajid Protective Mist Bodifier, 8 oz. for $8 at CVS (a better deal is to purchase the 32-oz. size for only $20 directly from Taliah Waajid's website, http://www.naturalhair.org/protectivemistbodifier32oz.asp x).

Moisturizers

Elasta QP Olive Oil and Mango Butter Moisturizer, 8¼ oz. for $3.99 at Walgreens;

Shea Moisture products, 12 oz. for $9.99 at Walgreens;

Fruit of the Earth 100% Aloe Vera Gel, 12 oz. for $3.97 at Walmart;

Luster S-Curl No Drip Activator, 8 oz. for $5 at CVS (or it may be cheaper at your local beauty supply store).

Google Tools

Don't buy another product online without following this advice! Instead of visiting numerous websites to comparison shop before making an online purchase, let Google do the footwork for you. Starting from the homepage of Google www.google.com, type the name of the product you are searching for into the search bar and hit enter. For example, let's use one of my all-time favorite conditioners, Aubrey Organics Honeysuckle Rose. Once the search results pop up, you should see a few pictures of the product (depending on its popularity), and a link that says "Shop for Aubrey Organics Honeysuckle Rose." Here is a screenshot:

Google and the Google logo are registered trademarks of Google Inc., used with permission.

Once you click the link that says "Shop for Aubrey Organics Honeysuckle Rose ... on Google," you should see a page that lists the prices of this product at locations near you. In order to have Google search your local stores, set your location. For example, I entered 30315 to tell Google that I am in Atlanta, GA.

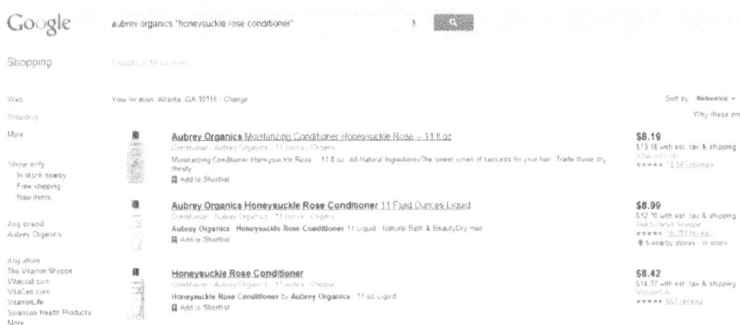

Google and the Google logo are registered trademarks of Google Inc., used with permission.

Looking at these shopping results from Google, I can see that with the cost of tax and shipping included, The Vitamin Shoppe has the best price for me to purchase the Aubrey Organics Honeysuckle Rose conditioner.

Now that I know the best place to purchase this specific conditioner online, what if I wanted to buy it locally? On the right-hand side of the screen, next to the first result, I see that Google has found five nearby stores that carry the Aubrey Organics Honeysuckle Rose conditioner. Better yet, Google has even checked the availability of the conditioner, and I can see that it is in stock at these stores.

Using its popular Map feature, Google pulls up a listing of the nearest places for me to purchase the Aubrey Organics conditioner. Not only does Google provide the address for each store, it also provides the phone number, the hours of operation, the cost, and information on stock availability. If any one of these locations had a stock status of "low", I would know to avoid that location, just in case they sold out before I got there.

While Google does not currently search the inventory of every store, I still appreciate its giving me helpful information about places near me that sell this hard-to-find product.

❦❦❦❦❦❦5❦❦❦❦❦❦❦
Go to the Source

This chapter focuses on teaching you how to skip the hair company middleman and save money by going directly to the wholesale source to purchase your hair products and accessories.

Satin Scarves

Have you ever gone to the beauty supply store to purchase a new satin scarf and flipped the package over to find out what the material was made of? No? Well, you should. Most of the scarves and hair wraps masquerading as satin are actually made of polyester. Do your natural hair a favor and head to your local fabric store to purchase a scarf-size piece of real satin. No need to take any measurements, just bring your favorite scarf and the fabric store clerk will be able to tell you how many yards of satin you need to make your own scarf. The best part? You won't even need to pick up a needle and thread. Just cut your scarf to your preferred size and call it a day.

Now, if you want to get fancy, while you are at the store purchase two yards of silk, a needle, and thread. Yes, ladies, I'm telling you to embrace your inner Martha Stewart by making your own satin pillowcases. This is one of the easiest sewing projects out there. Even if you've never heard of a thimble and never threaded a needle, you can do this.

1. Purchase two yards of satin fabric. Take it home and lay it on a clean floor or large table.

2. Lay one of your own standard-size pillowcases over the fabric. Using it as a guide, cut out two pieces of satin, making sure that each piece you cut is two to three inches longer and wider than your pillowcase. If you want your pillow to actually fit inside the pillowcase, don't skip this step!

3. Place the two pieces you've just cut on top of one another. If your satin is silky on only one side, make sure the fabric is lying with the silky sides touching each other.

4. Sew the two pieces together on the shortest side, then sew the two long sides of the pillowcase. Don't sew the remaining end. This is where you will insert the pillow.

5. Using the open end that you didn't sew, turn the fabric inside out, and *voila!* Instant satin pillowcase!

Your pillowcase doesn't have to be perfect. It's meant to be pleasing to the hair, not necessarily to the eye. Besides, by making your own satin pillowcase, you just slashed the cost by nearly 70%.

For additional savings, Joann fabric and craft stores are excellent local sources of satin that you can use for scarves or pillowcases, if you have them in your area. Save money by visiting http://www.joann.com/coupon/before your visit. The store usually offers a coupon good for 50% off any regularly-priced product.

Got Silk?

The company **Dharma Trading** (http://www.dharmatrading.com) imports high-quality, Grade A silk and sells it for prices that are unbelievably low, especially compared to what you would pay in a high-end store. If you are in the market for silk scarves, Dharma Trading sells scarves of all sizes from prices starting under $2 each. Once you visit the website and see the large variety of scarves available, it can be hard to determine which type of silk to buy and in what size. As a general guide, I suggest 21½ by 21½ inches if you have a small head and thin hair, or if you wear your hair straightened most of the time. This is approximately the same size as the colorful square bandanas you can find at your local beauty supply. I prefer to have a little bit more room, because I need my entire head to be covered, so I prefer the 35-by-35-inch size, which is a good choice for tying down thick natural hair. The black hand-rolled-hem 8mm Habotai scarf, sized 8 by 54 inches, is the perfect length for a gentle tie-on headband and is only $3.05. The 21½-by-21½-inch in black is $3.05, and the 35-by-35-inch scarf in white is $5.12. Prices are subject to change, but you can see that these prices for high-quality silk scarves are comparable to what you would pay for a fake satin head wrap from the beauty supply store, which typically retails for $2.99 to $3.99.

In addition to the scarves, check out their silk charmeuse pillowcases. They are a steal at only $12.65 each. Silk pillowcases are often sold for $25 each, so purchasing them directly from the wholesaler represents a savings of about 50%. Dharma Trading frequently runs special deals that allow you to choose a free gift when you make your first purchase. Currently, one of the free gifts on the list is a Habotai 8mm scarf. So you could actually end up purchasing two for the price of one.

Find Your Library Card

While we are on the subject of going directly to the source, don't forget about going to the book source: your local library. Hundreds of books are being published about natural hair, and although as an author it pains me to say this, you just can't purchase them all. Luckily for you, you don't have to. Instead of purchasing every book out there that's related to natural hair, save money by borrowing them from your friendly neighborhood library. Libraries have gotten pretty high-tech these days, and in addition to loaning the print copy of the book, many will let you borrow e-books in various formats.

So, how do you find out which books are available in your area without searching each library's catalog? I suggest using a website called WorldCat. WorldCat.org lets you search thousands of libraries for books on the topic of your choice. The best part is that WorldCat locates the book at libraries in your area and gives you the contact information you need to borrow the book.

If you need to access WorldCat from your cell phone, visit www.worldcat.org/m/ to find and search libraries on the mobile web. As an example, from the homepage of WorldCat.org, let's run a search using the phrase "natural hair":

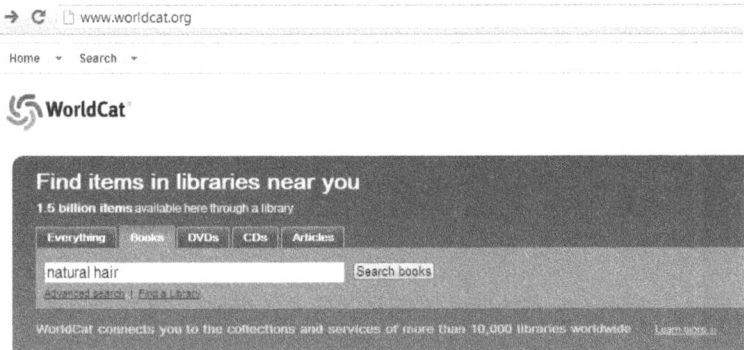

As shown in the screenshot below, the very first result is a natural hair-related book called "Textured tresses":

Since this book was published in 2004, let's run an advanced search to find books published in 2011 or later:

The results are as follows:

Now let's click on the first book listed, "Nappturosity," to get information on its availability in Tampa, Florida:

As you can see in the screenshot above, this book is available at two libraries within 25 miles of the location I entered.

That's how easy it is to use WorldCat to find books about natural hair that you can borrow from your local library for free.

Raw Ingredients and Bulk Bases

Have you ever wondered why some natural hair products are so expensive? Surely 100% pure shea butter doesn't really cost that much, right? Of course it doesn't! When you purchase products from hair companies, you are paying a premium for these goods. Hair care companies buy their raw materials and, in some cases, completely finished hair products from wholesalers at competitive prices. These companies then pass the costs of their fancy branded packaging, websites, and advertising on to their customers by charging much more for the product than they paid for it. Business is business, and that's just the way it works. But what if you could beat this system and make it work in your favor?

Many of the wholesale companies in the list below sell pre-made hair products, called bases, to companies which customize them by adding a few additional ingredients and then package and sell them as their own products. Many of these bases can be used as is, without further modification. So what does this have to do with saving money? Well, what if I told you that some of your favorite hair products were made with product bases that cost a fraction of the cost of the product itself?

Let's take the hypothetical company Pink's Kinks as an example. Let's say Pink's Kinks makes your favorite peppermint-fragranced deep conditioning hair treatment, but at $20 for an 8-oz. jar, it's out of your budget. Following Hair Commandment Number Three, you Google the top few ingredients in the product to see if you can find a cheaper alternative. To your surprise, you find a near-perfect match on the website of a wholesale company. What you just discovered is that Pink's Kink's didn't actually make that conditioner from scratch. Instead, the company purchased the base for the conditioner from the wholesale company and then simply added a small amount of peppermint essential oil to give it the wonderful scent you love. Well, guess what? You can do the same thing.

There are tons of wholesalers that sell product bases to the general public. In most cases, they offer various sizes and have no minimum purchase requirements, so you won't have to buy industrial-sized containers of their products.

Wholesale Suppliers of Hair Products

The following companies are wholesale suppliers of raw materials and natural hair-friendly ingredients, from common ingredients such as shea butter and aloe vera to more exotic oils and butters such as argan oil and murumuru butter.

Texas Natural Supply http://www.texasnaturalsupply.com sells high-quality herbs, botanicals, spices, essential oils, raw materials, and ingredients that can be used for making hair products. This is a great place to purchase hair butters. They have an extensive collection, including unrefined shea butter, whipped shea butter, shea aloe butter, avocado butter, mango butter, and green tea butter.

According to its website, **Bramble Berry** http://www.brambleberry.com "offers more than 2500 soap making products, including fragrance oils, soap molds, packaging, soap making kits, as well as supplies to make essential oils, lip butter flavorings, herbs and botanicals, cosmetics and much more."

Camden Grey http://www.camdengrey.com/ is one of the largest East Coast suppliers of aromatherapy and raw materials in the U.S.

Ingredients To Die For
http://www.ingredientstodiefor.com/ is a family-owned and -operated wholesale supplier of personal care ingredients and bases that prides itself on providing petro-, paraben-, formaldehyde-, artificial-color- and fragrance-free products.

From Nature With Love
http://www.fromnaturewithlove.com/ is a wholesale supplier of 1,750-plus natural ingredients used in bath, hair, and body products.

Wholesale Supplies Plus www.wholesalesuppliesplus.com offers a large variety of oils, butters, and essential oils. Popular offerings at the time of writing include apricot kernel oil, avocado oil, castor oil, coconut oil, glycerin, grapeseed oil, jojoba oil, olive oil, sweet almond oil, and wheat germ oil.

Essential Wholesale www.essentialwholesale.com has one of the largest selections of natural and organic unscented cosmetic bases in the world, as well as a huge selection of soap- and toiletry-making supplies. Several companies that market hair products to women with natural hair purchase their bases from this company, add a few drops of oil and fragrance, and charge three times the cost for their product. If you can do without the added fragrance or don't mind adding your own, you can get a steal of a deal by ordering directly from this wholesaler.

New Directions Aromatics http://www.newdirectionsaromatics.com/ is a leading wholesale supplier of 100% pure essential oils and provides a wide variety of hair-nourishing raw materials, such as silk amino acid and aloe vera gel juice.

Lotioncrafter http://www.lotioncrafter.com/ is a wholesale supplier of natural materials for the development of cosmetics and toiletries.

Mountain Rose Herbs http://mountainroseherbs.com/ offers an extensive selection of hair oils, hair butters, and herbal hair care products.

Duafe Naturals http://www.ujamaaessentials.com/ specializes in supplies and raw ingredients for the hair and skin. If you live in or near Bladensburg, Maryland, you can pick your order up directly from their warehouse.

Aquarius Aromatherapy and Soap Supplies http://www.aquariusaroma-soap.com/carries wholesale soap-making, cosmetic, spa, and personal care raw materials and packaging. Aquarius Aromatherapy orders are shipped from Mission, British Columbia, Canada, and they ship everywhere in North America, Europe, and Asia.

Creations from Eden http://www.creationsfromeden.com/ carries an extensive selection of high-quality raw ingredients, including nourishing butters, carrier oils, and essential oils, all of which are ethically sourced and free from harmful chemicals and pesticides.

Saffire Blue Inc. http://www.saffireblue.ca/ offers an extensive selection of high-quality cosmetic formulation supplies and shea butter, mango butter, and other exotic butters, as well as carrier oils, fragrance oils, cosmetic bases, cosmetic packaging, and clays. Orders are shipped from their offices in the U.S. and Canada. Bonus: order products online and pick them up directly from their warehouse in Courtland, Ontario, Canada.

Voyageur Soap http://www.voyageursoapandcandle.com sells hair care bases, such as a silk protein shampoo base and a hydrating daily conditioner, as well as aloe butter, shea butter, kokum butter, and an assortment of hair oils.

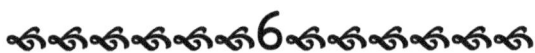

⬥⬥⬥⬥⬥⬥6⬥⬥⬥⬥⬥⬥⬥

Socialize

If you are an extrovert, one easy way to save money is to simply network with other women who have natural hair. Becoming a member of a natural hair community often comes with benefits such as group discounts, educational seminars, and the ability to do product swaps, all of which will help you save money and expand your circle of natural-haired friends.

Meetup.com is a website that helps groups of people with shared interests plan meetings and form offline clubs in local communities around the world. Go to www.meetup.com and do a search for natural hair. The site should automatically detect your location. If you want to search for groups in a different city, click the link to enter a new location. In the screenshot below, you can see that I searched for natural hair meetups in Washington, DC. The first meetup group, Simply FabULous Naturals and Transitioning, has 1,160 members.

When you join the group, you gain access to information about upcoming meetings, member profiles, and special discounts. While many groups are free, some charge an annual membership fee that usually costs less than ten dollars per year, which is worth it for the opportunity to connect with thousands of other natural women, attend fun educational and social events, and test out different hair goodies by doing product swaps with members.

Eventbrite.com is another website that allows you to find out about natural hair events in your area. While meetup.com focuses primarily on membership groups, Eventbrite focuses primarily on paid events, such as natural hair shows, seminars, and social events.

Natural Hair Shows

Attending natural hair shows is a good way to participate in seminars, sample hair products, and meet other women with natural hair. Many vendors who attend the shows offer great deals on the purchase of their products during the show. Keep in mind that while they are a lot of fun, attendance at natural hair shows is not free. The entry fee usually ranges from about $25 to $50, so make sure that you get your money's worth if you are planning on attending one. The website www.naturalhairshows.com provides a constantly updated listing of upcoming natural hair shows. You are bound to find some in your area.

Natural Hair Forums

If you have the time to peruse them, natural hair forums can be goldmines of free information about products, techniques, and other hair-related topics of interest. Many women post their personal experiences with hair products, pictures of their hair growth, and advice regarding styling and maintaining natural hair. Natural hair forums are a two-way street. Besides simply reading other people's testimonials, you can post your own testimonials, reviews, and questions to the community and get feedback from hundreds of other women with natural hair. Forums are an easy way for introverts to socialize with other women in a way that they might be less comfortable doing in person.

Here are a few popular natural hair forums:

The Long Hair Care Forum:
http://www.longhaircareforum.com

Black Hair Media:
http://forum.blackhairmedia.com/

Curly Nikki:
http://www.curlynikkiforums.com/

Naturally Curly:
http://www.naturallycurly.com/curltalk/

Nappturality:
http://www.nappturality.com/forum/forum.php

Glossary

If you haven't already noticed it, women on natural hair boards and blogs speak a language all their own. Just in case you don't speak "natural," I've included a handy list of popular terms and acronyms.

ACV: apple cider vinegar

APL: armpit-length hair

BC: big chop; cutting off all your chemically processed hair

BSL: bra-strap-length hair

BSS: beauty supply store

CL: chin-length hair

CBL: collarbone-length hair

Co-wash: conditioner wash; washing hair with conditioner rather than shampoo

Creamy Crack: a relaxer or perm

DC: deep condition

DIY: do it yourself

Dusting: a mini-trim; cutting off approximately ¼-inch of hair

EL: ear-length hair

EVOO: extra virgin olive oil

EVCO: extra virgin coconut oil

EO: essential oil

HHG: happy hair-growing

HIH: hand-in-hair disease

HIF: hand-in-fro disease

HL: hip-length hair

JBCO: Jamaican black castor oil

KCCC: Kinky Curly Curling Custard

LHCF: the website Long Hair Care Forum

MBL: Mid-back-length hair

NG: new growth

NL: neck-length hair

No poo: not using shampoo

PJ: product junkie; someone who buys a lot of hair products

Poo: shampoo

Pre-poo: conditioning the hair, usually with oils, prior to shampooing or conditioner washing

SL: shoulder-length hair

Slip: how easily a hair product, usually conditioner, allows a comb or your fingers to glide through the hair.

SLS: sodium lauryl sulfate; a chemical lathering agent found in many shampoos

SSK: single-strand knots

TWA: teeny-weeny Afro

WNG: wash and go

WSL: waist-length hair

A Note from the Author

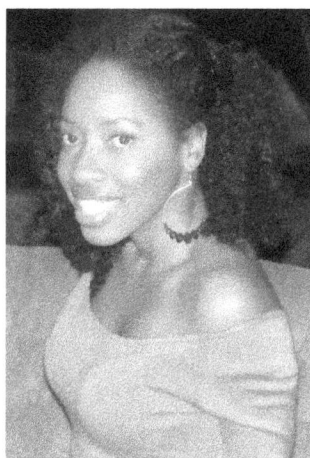

Dear Readers:

I hope that this book has been the wind beneath your natural hair wings, leading you to the highest peaks of financial savings!

In all seriousness, I truly hope that these tips will help you go (or stay!) natural without going broke.

Stop by my website www.mochamoolah.com for more information on my personal hair journey and to connect with me directly, I would love to hear from you! If you enjoyed this book, please spread the word by leaving a review and stay tuned for my upcoming works including the April 2013 release of "The Kinky Code: Unlocking the Secrets of Your Natural Hair".

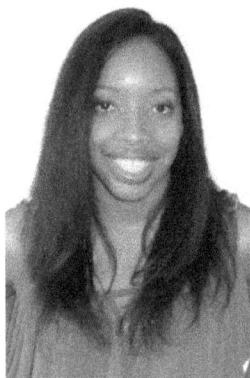

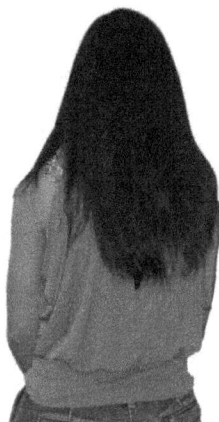